Renal Diet Simple & Delicious Recipes

Tasty and Affordable Renal Diet Recipes to Enjoy Your Diet and Boost Your Metabolism

Jacqueline Austin

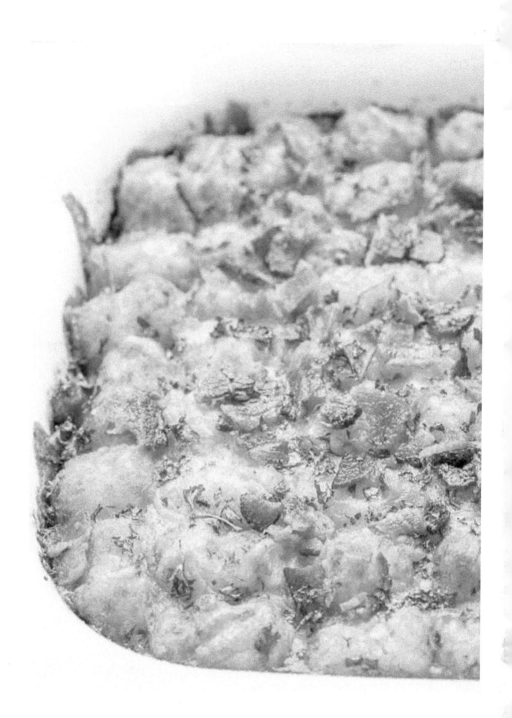

sources. Please consult a licensed professional before attempting any techniques outlined in this book.

By reading this document, the reader agrees that under no circumstances is the author responsible for any losses, direct or indirect, which are incurred as a result of the use of information contained within this document, including, but not limited to, — errors, omissions, or inaccuracies.

Table of Contents

Green Lettuce Bacon Breakfast Bake

Ingredients:

- 5 eggs

- 3 cups baby green lettuce, chopped

- 1 tbsp. olive oil

- 8 bacon slices, cooked and chopped

- 2 Red bell peppers, sliced

- 2 tbsp. chives, chopped

- Pepper

- Salt

Directions:

1. First, take a medium-sized baking dish and spray it with cooking spray and set aside; then preheat the oven to 350 F.
2. In a relatively large skillet, pour the oil and add the green lettuce, which should cook until wilted.

3. At this point, take a bowl and add the eggs, salt, and wilted green lettuce. Mix well.

4. Take the baking dish that we had previously set aside and pour the mixture together with the bacon, red peppers, and chives.

5. Let bake for 45 minutes and then serve.

Nutrition Facts Per Serving:

Calories: 273 kcal

Fat: 20.4 g

Carbohydrates: 3.1 g

Sugar: 1.7 g

Protein: 17 g

Cholesterol: 301 mg

Sodium: 720 mg

Potassium: 225 mg

Phosphorus: 161 mg

Healthy Green Lettuce Tomato Muffins

Preparation Time: 10 minutes

Cooking Time: 20 minutes

Servings: 12

Ingredients:

- 12 eggs

- 1/2 tsp. Italian seasoning

- 1 cup Red bell peppers, chopped

- 4 tbsp. water

- 1 cup fresh green lettuce, chopped

- ½ tsp pepper

- 1 tsp salt

Directions:

1. First, preheat the oven to 350 F and prepare a muffin tray by spraying the cooking spray.
2. Set the tray aside and move on to the actual preparation.

3. Next, take a mixing bowl and combine the eggs with water, Italian seasoning, pepper, and salt. Mix well, and then add the green lettuce and red peppers.
4. Take the muffin tray again and pour the mixture on top and bake for 20 minutes.
5. Serve.

Nutrition Facts Per Serving:

Calories: 67 kcal

Fat: 4.5 g

Carbohydrates: 1 g

Sugars: 0.8 g

Protein: 5.7 g

Cholesterol: 164 mg

Sodium: 257 mg

Potassium: 94 mg

Phosphorus: 91.5 mg

Chicken Egg Breakfast Muffin

Preparation Time: 10 minutes

Cooking Time: 15 minutes

Servings: 12

Ingredients:

- 5 eggs

- 1 cup cooked chicken, chopped

- 3 tbsp. green onions, chopped

- ¼ tsp. garlic powder

- Pepper

- ½ Salt

Directions:

1. Start by getting a muffin tray and spraying cooking spray on it. Also, preheat the oven to 400 F.
2. Now, take a large bowl and combine the eggs with pepper, salt, and garlic powder and mix well.
3. Then add the rest of the ingredients, continuing to mix.

4. When the compote is ready, pour it into the muffin tray and bake for 15 minutes.
5. Serve.

Nutrition Facts Per Serving:

Calories: 571 kcal

Fat: 8 g

Carbohydrates: 0.4 g

Sugar: 0.3 g

Protein: 6.5 g

Cholesterol: 145 mg

Sodium: 91 mg

Potassium: 76.45 mg

Phosphorus: 88.86 mg

Breakfast Egg Salad

Preparation Time: 10 minutes

Cooking Time: 8 minutes

Servings: 6

Ingredients:

- 6 large eggs

- 1 tbsp. fresh dill, chopped

- 4 tbsp. lite mayonnaise

- Pepper

- Salt

Directions:

1. Start by preparing the boiled eggs.
2. Pour eggs into a pot with water and bring to a boil. Cook the eggs for 8 minutes when the water is boiling again.
3. Then, take a large bowl and combine all the ingredients. Stir well to even out all the flavors.
4. Serve.

Nutrition Facts Per Serving:

Calories: 140 kcal

Fat: 10 g

Carbohydrates: 4 g

Sugars: 1 g

Protein: 8 g

Cholesterol: 245 mg

Sodium: 474 mg

Phosphorus: 78 mg

Potassium: 64 mg

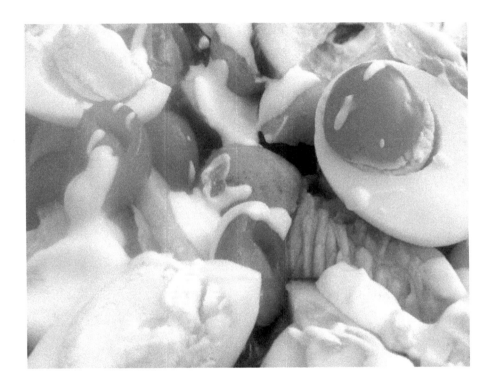

Healthy Vegetable Tofu Scramble

Preparation Time: 10 minutes

Cooking Time: 7 minutes

Servings: 2

Ingredients:

- 1/2 block firm tofu, crumbled

- 1/4 tsp. ground cumin

- 1 tbsp. turmeric

- 1 cup green lettuce

- 1/4 cup zucchini, chopped

- 1 tbsp. olive oil

- 1 tomato, chopped

- 1 tbsp. chives, chopped

- 1 tbsp. coriander, chopped

- Pepper

- 0.5-1 tsp salt

Directions:

1. Take a frying pan and pour over the oil. Let it heat for a few seconds over medium heat.
2. At this point, add the tomato, zucchini, and green lettuce. Let it fry for about 2 minutes.
3. After this time has elapsed, add the tofu, cumin, turmeric, salt, and pepper. Allow sautéing for another 5 minutes.
4. Season with chives and cilantro and serve.

Nutrition Facts Per Serving:

Calories: 115 kcal

Total Fat: 8.39 g

Carbs: 6.78 g

Sugars: 2.39 g

Protein: 3.72 g

Sodium: 18.04 mg

Potassium: 313 mg

Phosphorus: 41 mg

Cheese Coconut Pancake

Preparation Time: 10 minutes

Cooking Time: 8 minutes

Servings: 1

Ingredients:

- 2 eggs

- 1 packet stevia

- 1/2 tsp. cinnamon

- 2 oz. cream cheese

- 1 tbsp. coconut flour

- 1/2 tsp. vanilla

Directions:

1. First, take a bowl and combine all ingredients, whisking to make a smooth mixture. Help yourself with an immersion blender or whisk (it will take longer).

2. Then heat a skillet over medium-high heat, making sure to spray cooking spray on top.

3. At this point, pour the mixture into the hot skillet and cook until the first bubbles appear. At that point, flip

the pancake over and cook on the other side until it is slightly brown.

4. Remove from the skillet and serve piping hot.

Nutrition Facts Per Serving:

Calories: 181.91 kcal

Fat: 14.46 g

Carbohydrates: 5.54 g

Sugars: 1.88 g

Protein: 7.8 g

Cholesterol: 389 m

Potassium: 102 mg

Phosphorus: 117 mg

Sodium: 154.15 mg

Cheesy Scrambled Eggs with Fresh Herbs

Preparation Time: 10 minutes

Cooking Time: 5 minutes

Servings: 4

Ingredients:

- Eggs 3

- Egg whites 2

- Cream cheese 1/2 cup

- Unsweetened rice milk 1/4 cup

- Chopped scallion 1 Tbsp. green part only

- Chopped fresh tarragon 1 Tbsp.

- Unsalted butter 2 tsp.

- Ground black pepper to taste

Directions:

1. Take a bowl and combine the whole eggs and the egg whites, cream cheese, rice milk, scallion, and tarragon. Mix until smooth and homogeneous.

19

2. At this point, place the butter in a skillet and let it melt over low heat.
3. Once the butter is melted, add the egg mixture and cook for 5 minutes, taking care to stir, until the eggs are cooked, and everything is creamy.
4. Finish with pepper and serve.

Nutrition Facts Per Serving:

Calories: 221 kcal

Fat: 19 g

Carbs: 3 g

Phosphorus: 119 mg

Potassium: 140 mg

Sodium: 193 mg

Protein: 8 g

Coconut Breakfast Smoothie

Preparation Time: 5 minutes

Cooking Time: 0 minutes

Servings: 1

Ingredients:

- 1/4 cup whey protein powder

- 1/2 cup coconut milk

- 5 drops liquid stevia

- 1 tbsp. coconut oil

- 1 tsp. vanilla

- 2 tbsp. coconut butter

- 1/4 cup water

- 1/2 cup ice

Directions:

1. Attach all ingredients into the blender and blend until smooth.
2. Serve and enjoy.

Nutrition Facts Per Serving:

Calories: 560 kcal

Fat: 45 g

Carbohydrates: 12 g

Sugar: 4 g

Protein: 25 g

Cholesterol: 60 mg

Sodium: 41.5 mg

Potassium: 153 mg

Phosphorus: 91.5 mg

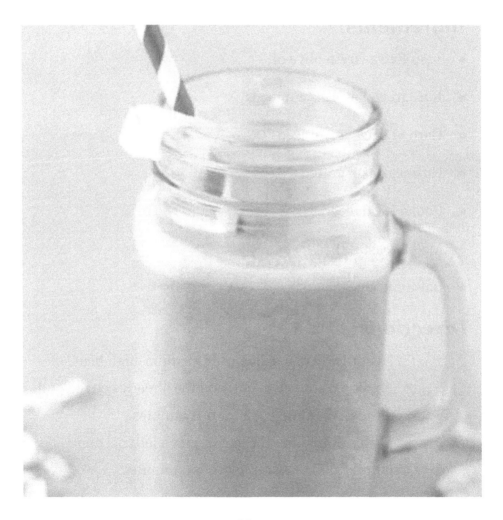

Turkey and Green Lettuce Scramble on Melba Toast

Preparation Time: 2 minutes

Cooking Time: 14 minutes

Servings: 2

Ingredients:

- 1 tsp Extra virgin olive oil

- Raw green lettuce 1 cup

- Garlic 1/2 clove, minced

- Nutmeg 1 tsp. grated

- Cooked and diced turkey breast 1 cup

- Melba toast 2 slices

- Balsamic vinegar 1 tsp.

Directions:

1. Heat the oil in a skillet over medium-high heat.
2. As soon as the oil is hot, add the already cooked and diced turkey and cook for 6-8 minutes.
3. At this point, add the garlic, green lettuce, and nutmeg and cook for another 6 minutes.

4. Place the Melba Toast on a plate and add the turkey and green lettuce as soon as they are ready.
5. Drizzle with balsamic vinegar and serve.

Nutrition Facts Per Serving:

Calories: 301 kcal

Fat: 19 g

Carb: 12 g

Phosphorus: 215 mg

Potassium: 269 mg

Sodium: 360 mg

Protein: 19 g

Vegetable Healthy Omelet

Preparation Time: 15 minutes

Cooking Time: 10 minutes

Servings: 3

Ingredients:

- Egg whites 4

- Egg 1

- Chopped fresh parsley 2 Tbsps.

- Water 2 Tbsps.

- Olive oil spray

- Chopped and boiled red bell pepper 1/2 cup

- Chopped scallion 1/4 cup, both green and white parts

- Ground black pepper

Directions:

1. First, take a bowl and combine the egg along with the egg whites and water. Whisk the mixture until all the ingredients are well blended.

2. Separately, heat a skillet over medium heat with cooking spray.

3. As soon as the skillet is hot, pour in the peppers and shallots, and sauté for 3 minutes until they have reached a morbid consistency.
4. At this point, pour the egg mixture into the skillet and cook until they have reached a thick consistency.
5. Season with black pepper and serve.

Nutrition Facts Per Serving:

Calories: 112.82 kcal

Fat: 6.36 g

Carbs: 4.22 g

Sugars: 2.37 g

Phosphorus: 68.8 mg

Potassium: 250 mg

Sodium: 132.89 mg

Protein: 9.81 g

Mexican Style Burritos

Preparation Time: 5 minutes

Cooking Time: 15 minutes

Servings: 2

Ingredients:

- Olive oil 1 Tbsp.

- 2 Corn tortillas

- Red onion 1/4 cup, chopped

- Red bell peppers 1/4 cup, chopped

- Red chili 1/2, deseeded and chopped

- Eggs 2

- Juice of 1 lime

- Cilantro 1 Tbsp. chopped

Directions:

1. Heat a grill over medium heat and arrange the tortillas. Let them heat for 1 to 2 minutes on each side until lightly toasted.

2. Meanwhile, take a skillet and sauté the onion along with the red chili and afterward add the peppers and cook for 5 0 6 minutes, until soft.

3. Also, add the eggs to the skillet and cook for another 10 minutes until the eggs are fully cooked.
4. Divide the egg and vegetable mixture between the two tortillas, sprinkle with cilantro and lime juice and serve.

Nutrition Facts Per Serving:

Calories: 202 kcal

Fat: 13 g

Carb: 19 g

Phosphorus: 184 mg

Potassium: 233 mg

Sodium: 77 mg

Protein: 9 g

Healthy Bulgur, Couscous and Buckwheat Cereal

Preparation Time: 10 minutes

Cooking Time: 25 minutes

Servings: 4

Ingredients:

- Water 2 1/4 cups

- Vanilla rice milk 1 1/4 cups

- Uncooked bulgur 6 Tbsps.

- Uncooked whole buckwheat 2 Tbsps.

- Sliced apple 1 cup

- Plain uncooked couscous 6 Tbsps.

- Ground cinnamon 1/2 tsp.

Directions:

1. Fill a saucepan with the water and milk and bring to a boil over medium heat. Once it comes to a boil, add the bulgur, apple, buckwheat, and couscous.

2. At this point, lower the heat and simmer for 20-25 minutes, taking care to stir occasionally.

3. As soon as bulgur is tender and grains are cooked, remove the saucepan from heat, add cinnamon and stir again. Finally, let everything rest with the lid on.
4. Before serving, be sure to stem the grains with a fork.

Nutrition Facts Per Serving:

Calories: 347.54 kcal

Fat: 2.45 g

Carbs: 74.22 g

Sugars: 13.94 g

Phosphorus: 260 mg

Potassium: 308 mg

Sodium: 71.75 mg

Protein: 9.35 g

Sweet Pancakes

Preparation Time: 10 minutes

Cooking Time: 4 minutes

Servings: 5

Ingredients:

- 1 cup All-purpose flour

- 1 Tbsp Granulated sugar

- 2 Tsps. Baking powder.

- 2 Egg whites

- 1 cup Unsweetened Almond milk

- 2 Tbsps. Olive oil

- 1 Tbsp Maple extract

Directions:

1. Take two bowls and mix the flour, sugar, and baking powder in one bowl; in another, the egg whites, milk, oil, and maple extract.

2. At this point, take the bowl with the flour mixture and make a well in the center and pour the egg

mixture into it, making sure to stir, so you get a smooth, even batter.

3. Next, take a non-stick skillet and heat it on the stove. Then, pour in 1/5 of the batter, and cook the first pancake for 2 minutes on each side.

4. Repeat the same process with the remaining batter to make the other pancakes.

5. Serve.

Nutrition Facts Per Serving:

Calories: 445.04 kcal

Fat: 16.27 g

Carbs: 64.08 g

Sugars: 14.8 g

Phosphorus: 183.6 mg

Potassium: 180.2 mg

Sodium: 619.89 mg

Protein: 10.17 g

Breakfast Smoothie

Preparation Time: 15 minutes

Cooking Time: 0 minutes

Servings: 2

Ingredients:

- Frozen blueberries 1/2 cup

- Pineapple chunks 1/2 cup

- English cucumber 1/2 cup

- Apple 1/2

- Water 1/2 cup

Directions:

1. Put the pineapple, blueberries, cucumber, apple, and water in a blender and blend until thick and smooth.
2. Pour into 2 glasses and serve.

Nutrition Facts Per Serving:

Calories: 87 kcal

Fat: 0.4 g

Carbs: 22 g

Phosphorus: 28 mg

Potassium: 192 mg

Sodium: 3 mg

Protein: 0.7 g

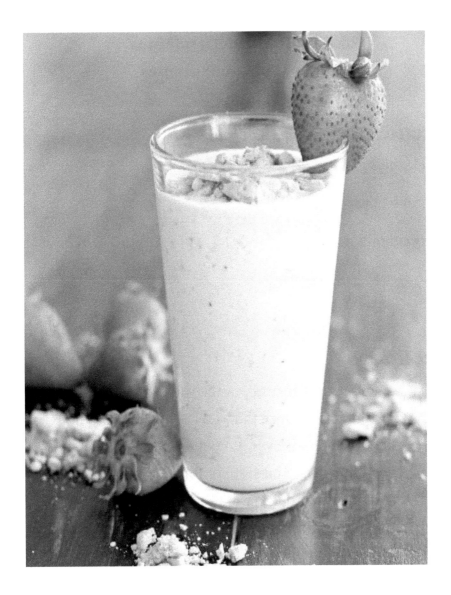

Buckwheat and Grapefruit Porridge

Preparation Time: 5 minutes
Cooking Time: 20 minutes

Servings: 2

Ingredients:

- Buckwheat 1/2 cup

- Water 2 cups

- Almond milk 1 1/2 cups

- Grapefruit –1/4, chopped

- Honey 1 Tbsp.

Directions:

1. Take a saucepan and put the water to boil over medium heat. Once the water is boiling, add the buckwheat and cover the pot with the lid.

2. Lower the heat and simmer for 7-10 minutes, making sure the water doesn't dry out.

3. As soon as most of the water is absorbed, turn off the stove and set it aside for 5 minutes.

4. Drain the excess water from the saucepan and add the almond milk, stirring and heating for 5 minutes.

5. Add the honey and grapefruit.

6. Serve.

Nutrition Facts per Serving:

Calories: 231 kcal

Fat: 4 g

Carbs: 43 g

Phosphorus: 165 mg

Potassium: 370 mg

Sodium: 135 mg

Egg and Veggie Muffins

Preparation Time: 15 minutes

Cooking Time: 20 minutes

Servings: 4

Ingredients:

- 1 puff cooking oil spray

- Eggs 4

- Unsweetened rice milk 2 Tbsp.

- Sweet onion 1/2, chopped

- Red bell pepper 1/2, chopped

- a sprig of parsley

- Pinch red pepper flakes

- Pinch ground black pepper

Directions:

1. First, be sure to preheat the oven to 350F.
2. Next, take four muffin pans and spray with cooking spray. Set aside.

3. In a bowl, combine the milk, eggs, onion, red bell pepper, parsley, red bell pepper flakes, and black pepper and mix well.
4. Pour the egg mixture into the previously prepared muffin pans and bake for about 10-20 minutes until the muffins are puffy and golden brown.
5. Serve.

Nutrition Facts per Serving:

Calories: 184 kcal

Fat: 5 g

Carbs: 3 g

Phosphorus: 110 mg

Potassium: 117 mg

Sodium: 75 mg

Protein: 7 g

Chicken and Mushroom Stew

Preparation Time: 10 minutes

Cooking Time: 35 minutes

Servings: 4

Ingredients:

- 2 chicken breast halves

- 1 pound mushrooms, sliced (5-6 cups)

- 1 bunch spring onion, chopped

- 4 tablespoons olive oil

- 1 teaspoon thyme

- Salt and pepper as needed

Directions:

1. First, heat the oil in a large deep pan over medium-high heat.
2. After that, add the chicken and cook for 4-5 minutes per side until lightly browned.
3. At this point, add the spring onions and mushrooms and season with salt and pepper, depending on your taste.
4. Next, mix well and then put the lid on and bring to a boil.

5. Lower the heat and simmer for 25 minutes.

6. Serve.

Nutrition Facts Per Serving:

Calories: 850.36 kcal

Fat: 58.04 g

Carbohydrates: 10.79 g

Sugars: 5.54 g

Protein: 72.49 g

Sodium: 214.45 mg

Potassium: 1530.13 mg

Phosphorus: 750 mg

Roasted Carrot Soup

Preparation Time: 10 minutes

Cooking Time: 45 minutes

Servings: 4

Ingredients:

- 8 large carrots, washed and peeled

- 6 tablespoons olive oil

- 1-quart broth

- Cayenne pepper to taste

- Salt and pepper to taste

Directions:

1. First, preheat the oven to 425 F.
2. Then, on a baking sheet, add the carrots and drizzle them with olive oil. Bake the carrots and let them cook for 30-45 minutes.
3. After the carrots are cooked, place them in a blender and add the broth. Then, blend and reduce to a puree.
4. Heat the puree in a saucepan and season with salt, pepper, and cayenne.

5. Drizzle with olive oil and serve.

Nutrition Facts per Serving:

Calories: 510.8 kcal

Fat: 43.92 g

Carbohydrates: 29.55 g

Sugars: 14.8 g

Protein: 3.81 g

Sodium: 2239.24 mg

Potassium: 916 mg

Phosphorus: 106 mg

Healthy Garlic and Butter-flavored Cod

Preparation Time: 5 minutes

Cooking Time: 20 minutes

Servings: 3

Ingredients:

- 3 Cod fillets, 8 ounces each

- 3/4 pound baby bok choy halved

- 1/3 cup almond butter, thinly sliced

- 1 1/2 tablespoons garlic, minced

- Salt and pepper to taste

Directions:

1. First, preheat the oven to 400 F.
2. Take some aluminum foil and cut out three sheets (large enough to fit the fillet).
3. Lay the cod fillet on each sheet and add the butter and garlic on top.
4. After that, add the bok choy and season with pepper and salt.
5. Fold the aluminum foil over and create pouches to place on a baking sheet. Then, bake for 20 minutes.

43

6. After these minutes are up, place the bags with the cod on a cooling rack and allow them to cool.

7. Serve.

Nutrition Facts per Serving:

Calories: 554.78 kcal

Fat: 25.53 g

Carbohydrates: 14.72 g

Protein: 72.46 g

Sodium: 897.07 mg

Potassium: 318.49 mg

Phosphorus: 212.52 mg

Healthy Tilapia Broccoli Platter

Preparation Time: 4 minutes

Cooking Time: 15 minutes

Servings: 2

Ingredients :

- 6 ounces of tilapia, frozen

- 1 cup of broccoli florets, fresh

- 1 teaspoon of lemon pepper seasoning

- 1 tablespoon of almond butter

- 1 tablespoon of garlic, minced

Directions:

1. First, preheat the oven to 350 F.
2. Then, add fish in foil packets and arrange broccoli around the fish.
3. After that, sprinkle with lemon pepper and close the packets, sealing well.
4. Allow cooking for about 15 minutes.
5. Meanwhile, in a bowl, add the garlic and butter, mix well and keep the mixture aside.
6. Remove the packets from the oven and transfer them to a serving dish.

7. Place the butter on top of the fish and broccoli, serve and enjoy!

Nutrition Facts per Serving:

Calories: 146.99 kcal

Fat: 5.92 g

Carbohydrates: 2 g

Protein: 19.72 g

Sodium: 305.44 mg

Potassium: 400 mg

Phosphorus: 200 mg

Parsley Scallops

Preparation Time: 5 minutes

Cooking Time: 25 minutes

Servings: 4

Ingredients:

- 16 large sea scallops

- 1 1/2 tablespoons olive oil

- Salt and pepper to taste

- 8 tablespoons almond butter

- 2 garlic cloves, minced

Directions:

1. In a skillet, add the oil and heat over medium heat. Meanwhile, Season the scallops with salt and pepper.

2. Once the oil is hot, sauté the scallops for 2 minutes on each side and repeat the same process with all the scallops. Once cooked, remove the scallops from the pan and add the butter to the pan to melt.

3. Add the garlic and cook for 15 minutes.

4. Return the scallops to the pan and stir to coat.

5. Serve and enjoy!

Nutrition Facts per Serving:

Calories: 409 kcal

Fat: 24.91 g

Carbohydrates: 13.36 g

Protein: 34 g

Sodium: 1382.42 mg

Potassium: 600 mg

Phosphorus: 900 mg

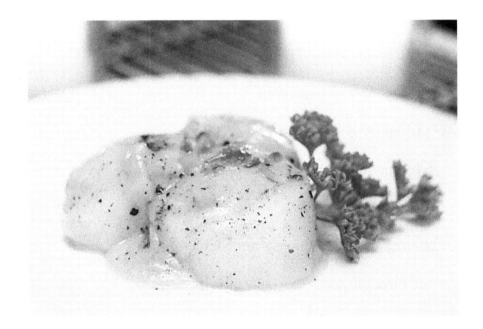

Blackened Chicken

Preparation Time: 10 minutes

Cooking Time: 10 minutes

Servings: 4

Ingredients:

- 1/2 teaspoon paprika

- 1/8 teaspoon salt

- 1/4 teaspoon cayenne pepper

- 1/4 teaspoon ground cumin

- 1/4 teaspoon dried thyme

- 1/8 teaspoon ground white pepper

- 1/8 teaspoon onion powder

- 2 chicken breasts, boneless and skinless

- 2 tsp. olive oil

Directions:

1. First, grease a baking sheet and preheat the oven to 350 F.
2. Take a cast-iron skillet and heat ½ tsp. of oil for 5 minutes on high heat.

3. Meanwhile, take a small bowl and mix salt, paprika, cumin, white pepper, cayenne, thyme, onion powder.
4. Then, oil the chicken breast on both sides and coat the breast with the spice mix.
5. Transfer the chicken to the hot pan and cook for 1 minute per side.
6. Transfer to the prepared baking sheet and bake for 5 minutes.
7. Serve and enjoy!

Nutrition Facts per Serving:

Calories: 136 kcal

Fat: 5 g

Carbohydrates: 1 g

Protein: 44 g

Potassium: 690 mg

Phosphorus: 430 mg

Sodium: 240 mg

Spicy Paprika Lamb Chops

Preparation Time: 10 minutes

Cooking Time: 10 minutes

Servings: 4

Ingredients:

- 0.5 lb. lamb racks, cut into chops

- Salt and pepper to taste

- 3 tablespoons paprika

- 3/4 cup cumin powder

- 1 teaspoon chili powder

Directions:

1. Mix the paprika, cumin, chili, salt, and pepper inside a bowl.
2. Add the lamb chops and allow the spice mixture to adhere to the lamb.
3. Heat a grill to medium temperature and add the lamb chops; cook for 5 minutes.
4. Turn and cook for another 5 minutes.
5. Serve and enjoy!

Nutrition Facts Per Serving:

Calories: 529.25 kcal

Fat: 37.34 g

Carbohydrates: 22.7 g

Protein: 108.72 g

Sodium: 585.4 mg

Potassium: 600 mg

Phosphorus: 400 mg

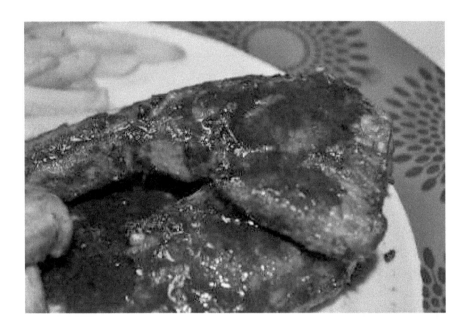

Healthy Mushroom and Olive Sirloin Steak

Preparation Time: 10 minutes

Cooking Time: 14 minutes

Servings: 4

Ingredients:

- 1 pound boneless beef sirloin steak

- 1 large red onion, chopped

- 1 cup mushrooms

- 4 garlic cloves, thinly sliced

- 4 tablespoons olive oil

- 1 cup parsley leaves, finely cut

Directions:

1. Heat 2 tbsp. oil over medium-high heat in a large skillet.
2. Add the beef and cook until both sides are browned; remove the beef from the skillet and discard the fat.
3. At this point, add the rest of the oil to the skillet and heat it.

4. Add the onions and garlic and cook for 2-3 minutes, stirring well.

5. Return the beef to the skillet and lower the heat to medium.

6. Cook for 3-4 minutes with the lid on.

7. Garnish with parsley.

8. Serve and enjoy!

Nutrition Facts Per Serving:

Calories: 754.46 kcal

Fat: 57.82 g

Carbohydrates: 8.09 g

Sugars: 3 g

Protein: 49.58 g

Sodium: 140.58 mg

Potassium: 1168.62 mg

Phosphorus: 512 mg

Healthy Parsley and Chicken Breast

Preparation Time: 10 minutes

Cooking Time: 30 minutes

Servings: 4

Ingredients:

- 1 tablespoon dry parsley

- 1 tablespoon dry basil

- 4 chicken breast halves, boneless and skinless

- 1 garlic clove, sliced

- 1/2 teaspoon salt

- 1/2 teaspoon red pepper flakes, crushed

Directions:

1. First, preheat your oven to 350 F and prepare a 9x13-inch baking dish by greasing it with cooking spray.

2. Sprinkle one teaspoon parsley and one teaspoon basil on the baking sheet and arrange the chicken breast halves, spreading the garlic slices on top.

3. Take a small bowl and add one teaspoon parsley, one teaspoon basil, salt, red pepper, and mix well. Pour mixture over chicken breast.

4. Bake for 30 minutes.

5. Serve and enjoy!

Nutrition Facts Per Serving:

Calories: 560.55 kcal

Fat: 8 g

Carbohydrates: 0.4 g

Sugars: 0.7 g

Protein: 80.38 g

Sodium: 675.6 mg

Potassium: 734.35 mg

Phosphorus: 430 mg

Simple Mustard Chicken

Preparation Time: 10 minutes

Cooking Time: 35 minutes

Servings: 4

Ingredients:

- 3 chicken breasts

- 1/2 cup chicken broth

- 3-4 tablespoons mustard

- 2 tablespoons olive oil

- 1 teaspoon paprika

- 1 teaspoon chili powder

- 1 teaspoon garlic powder

Directions:

1. Combine the mustard, olive oil, paprika, chicken broth, garlic powder, chili powder in a small bowl to create an emulsion.
2. At this point, pour the emulsion over the chicken breasts and let marinate for 30 minutes.
3. Line a large baking sheet with parchment paper and arrange the chicken.
4. Bake for 35 minutes at 375 F

5. Serve and enjoy!

Nutrition Facts Per Serving:

Calories: 750 kcal

Fat: 80 g

Carbohydrates: 2 g

Protein: 130 g

Potassium: 1410.51 mg

Phosphorus: 1106.42 mg

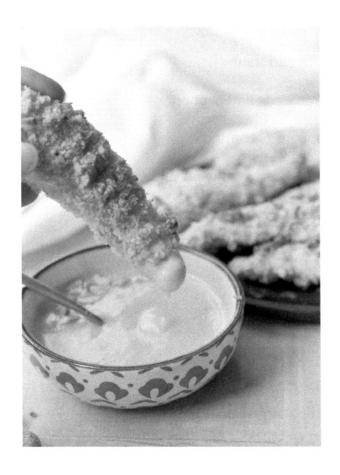

Healthy Golden Eggplant Fries

Preparation Time: 10 minutes

Cooking Time: 15 minutes

Servings: 8

Ingredients:

- 2 eggs

- 2 cups almond flour

- Sunflower seeds and pepper

- 2 tablespoons coconut oil, spray

- 2 eggplants, peeled and cut thinly

Directions:

1. First, preheat the oven to 400 degrees F.
2. Next, mix the almond flour with the sunflower seeds and black pepper in a bowl.
3. Separately, beat the eggs in another bowl until frothy.
4. Dip the eggplant pieces into the eggs and toss them in the flour mixture.
5. Next, dip the eggplant again, first in the egg and then in the flour.

6. Take a baking sheet, grease it with coconut oil on top and arrange the eggplants.
7. Bake for about 15 minutes.
8. Serve.

Nutrition Facts Per Serving:

Calories: 855.72 kcal

Total Fat: 69.01 g

Carbs: 42.53 g

Sugars: 16.86 g

Protein: 30.63 g

Sodium: 69.88 mg

Potassium: 1543.09 mg

Phosphorus: 200.82 mg

Very Wild Mushroom Pilaf

Note: To make this recipe, a Slow Cooker is needed; alternatively, a Dutch oven or any heavy-duty pot with a good lid will work.

Preparation Time: 10 minutes

Cooking Time: 3 hours

Servings: 4

Ingredients:

- 1 cup wild rice
- 2 garlic cloves, minced
- 6 green onions, chopped
- 2 tablespoons olive oil
- 1/2 pound baby Bella mushrooms
- 2 cups water

Directions using Slow Cooker:

1. Add rice, garlic, onion, oil, mushrooms and water to your Slow Cooker.
2. Stir well until mixed.
3. Set the lid and cook on LOW for 3 hours.
4. Stir pilaf and divide between serving platters.
5. Enjoy!

Directions using other pots:

1. Sauté the oil in your pot along with the garlic and onion. Once the onion is nicely browned, add the mushrooms and cook for a few minutes. At that point, add the rice and let it blanch.
2. In the meantime, have the water heated in another small pot.
3. Once the rice has taken on some color, gradually pour the hot water into the pot and continue stirring until the rice is fully cooked. This will take about 30 minutes.
4. Serve.

Nutrition Facts Per Serving:

Calories: 210 kcal

Fat: 7 g

Carbohydrates: 16 g

Protein: 4 g

Phosphorus: 110 mg

Potassium: 117 mg

Sodium: 75 mg

Sporty Baby Carrots

Preparation Time: 5 minutes

Cooking Time: 5 minutes

Servings: 4

Ingredients:

- 1-pound baby carrots

- 1 cup water

- 1 tablespoon clarified ghee

- 1 tablespoon chopped up fresh mint leaves

- Sea flavored vinegar as needed

Directions :

1. Set a steamer rack on top of your pot and add the carrots.
2. Add water.
3. Lock the lid and cook at HIGH pressure for 2 minutes. Do a quick release.
4. Pass the carrots through a strainer and drain them.
5. Wipe the insert clean.
6. Set the insert to the pot and set the pot to Sauté mode.
7. Add clarified butter and allow it to melt.

8. Add mint and sauté for 30 seconds.
9. Add carrots to the insert and sauté well.
10. Remove them and sprinkle a bit of flavored vinegar on top.
11. Enjoy!

Nutrition Facts Per Serving:

Calories: 131 kcal

Fat: 10 g

Carbohydrates: 11 g

Protein: 1 g

Sodium: 85 mg

Phosphorus: 130 mg

Potassium: 147 mg

Saucy Garlic Greens

Preparation Time: 5 minutes

Cooking Time: 20 minutes

Servings: 4

Ingredients:

- 1/2 cup cashews

- 1/4 cup water

- 1 tablespoon lemon juice

- 1 teaspoon coconut aminos

- 1 clove peeled whole clove

- 1/8 teaspoon of flavored vinegar

- 1 bunch of leafy greens

- lite Sauce

Directions:

1. Drain and discard the soaking water from your cashews and add them to a blender to make the sauce.
2. Add fresh water, lemon juice, flavored vinegar, coconut aminos, and garlic.
3. Blend to obtain a smooth cream and transfer to a bowl.

4. Add 1/2 cup of water to the pot and place a steamer basket on it.
5. Add the greens to the basket.
6. Lock the lid and steam for 1 minute. Quick release the pressure.
7. Transfer the steamed greens to a strainer and extract excess water.
8. Place the greens into a mixing bowl.
9. Add lemon, garlic, sauce and toss.
10. Serve.

Nutrition Facts Per Serving:

Calories: 196.65 kcal

Fat: 15.88 g

Carbohydrates: 11.2 g

Sugars: 1.72 g

Protein: 5.25 g

Phosphorus: 167.87 mg

Potassium: 193.57 mg

Sodium: 5.48 mg

Pasta with Creamy Broccoli Sauce

Preparation Time: 15 minutes

Cooking Time: 40 minutes

Servings: 2

Ingredients:

- 1 tbsp. olive oil

- 0.25 lb. broccoli florets

- 1 1/2 garlic cloves, halved

- 1/2 cup low-sodium vegetable broth

- 1/4 cup whole-wheat spaghetti pasta

- 2 tbsp cream cheese

- 1/2 tsp. dried basil leaves

Directions:

1. Take a pot and set water to a boil to cook your pasta.
2. Meanwhile, put olive oil in a large skillet and sauté the broccoli with the garlic for 3 minutes.
3. Then, add the broth to the skillet and bring it to a simmer. Reduce the heat to low, partially cover the

skillet, and simmer until the broccoli is tender; it will take about 5–6 minutes.

4. Cook the pasta according to package directions or for 12 minutes. Drain when al dente, reserving 1 cup pasta water.

5. When the broccoli is tender, add the cream cheese, basil, and purée using an immersion blender.

6. Put the mixture into a food processor, about half at a time, and purée until smooth; then, transfer the sauce back into the skillet.

7. Add the cooked pasta to the broccoli sauce. Toss, adding enough pasta water until the sauce coats the pasta thoroughly. Serve

Nutrition Facts Per Serving:

Calories: 410 kcal

Fats: 26 g

Carbs: 36 g

Protein: 11 g

Sodium: 260 mg

Potassium: 900 mg

Phosphorus: 223 mg

Delicious Vegetarian Lasagna

Preparation time: 10 minutes

Cooking time: 1 ¼ hour

Servings: 4

Ingredients:

- 1 teaspoon basil

- 1 tablespoon olive oil

- 1/2 sliced red pepper

- 2 lasagna sheets

- 1/2 diced red onion

- 1/4 teaspoon black pepper

- 1 cup rice milk

- 1 minced garlic clove

- 1 cup sliced eggplant

- 1/2 sliced zucchini

- 1/2 pack soft tofu

- 1 teaspoon oregano

Directions:

1. Preheat the oven to 325f. or if gas, mark 3.
2. Slice zucchini, eggplant and pepper into vertical strips.
3. Add the rice milk and tofu to a food processor and blitz until smooth. Set aside.
4. Warm up the oil and add the onions and garlic for 3-4 minutes or until soft.
5. Sprinkle in the herbs (oregano) and pepper and allow to stir through for 5-6 minutes until hot.
6. Into a lasagna or suitable oven dish, layer 1 lasagna sheet, then 1/3 the eggplant, followed by 1/3 zucchini, then 1/3 pepper before pouring over 1/3 of tofu white sauce.
7. Repeat for the next 2 layers, finishing with the white sauce.
8. Add to the oven for 40-50 minutes or until the veg is soft and can easily be sliced into servings.

Nutrition Facts Per Serving:

Calories: 235 kcal

Protein: 5 g

Carbs: 10 g

Fat: 9 g

Sodium: 35 mg

Potassium: 129 mg

Phosphorus: 66 mg4

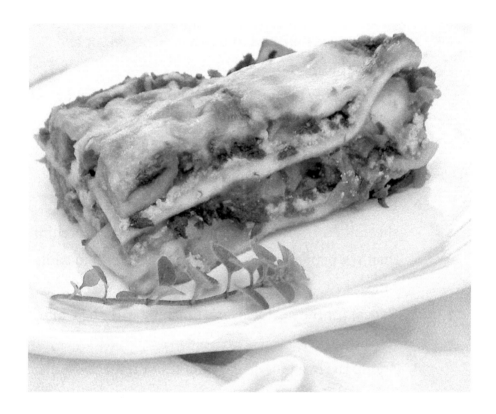

Creamy Pesto Pasta

Preparation time: 10 minutes

Cooking time: 20 minutes

Servings: 4

Ingredients:

- 4 ounces linguine noodles

- 2 cups packed basil leaves

- 2 cups packed arugula leaves

- 1/3 cup walnut pieces

- 3 garlic cloves

- 3 tbsp. extra-virgin olive oil

- Freshly ground black pepper

Directions:

1. Set a medium stock pot halfway with water, and bring to a boil. Cook the noodles al dente, for about 10-12 minutes and drain.

2. In a food processor, add the basil, arugula, walnuts, and garlic. Process until coarsely ground. With the

food processor running, slowly add the olive oil, and continue to mix until creamy. Season with pepper.

3. Merge the noodles with the pesto and serve.

Nutrition Facts Per Serving:

Calories: 394 kcal

Total Fat: 21 g

Saturated Fat: 3 g

Cholesterol: 0 mg

Carbohydrates: 0 g

Fiber: 3 g

Protein: 10 g

Phosphorus: 54 mg

Potassium: 148 mg

Sodium: 4 mg

Garden Salad

Preparation Time: 5 minutes

Cooking Time: 20 minutes

Servings: 4

Ingredients:

- 5 oz. raw peanuts in shell

- 1 bay leaf

- 1 medium-sized chopped up Red bell peppers

- 5 tablespoons, 1 teaspoon diced up green pepper

- 5 tablespoons, 1 teaspoon diced up sweet onion

- 2 tablespoons, 2 teaspoons finely diced hot pepper

- 2 tablespoons, 2 teaspoons diced up celery

- 1 tablespoon, 1 teaspoon olive oil

- 0.5 teaspoon flavored vinegar

- 1/4 teaspoon freshly ground black pepper

Directions:

1. Boil your peanuts for 1 minute and rinse them.
2. Their skin will be soft, so discard the skin.
3. Attach 2 cups of water to the Instant Pot.

4. Add bay leaf and peanuts.
5. Lock the lid and cook on HIGH pressure for 20 minutes. Drain the water.
6. Take a large bowl and add the peanuts, diced up vegetables.
7. Whisk in olive oil, lemon juice, pepper in another bowl.
8. Stream the mixture over the salad and mix!
9. Enjoy!

Nutrition Facts Per Serving:

Calories: 240 kcal

Fat: 4 g

Carbohydrates: 24 g

Protein: 5 g

Phosphorus: 110 mg

Potassium: 117 mg

Sodium: 75 mg

Zucchini Pasta

Preparation Time: 15 minutes

Cooking Time: 30 Minutes

Servings: 4

Ingredients:

- 3 Tablespoons of olive oil

- 2 Cloves garlic, minced

- 3 Zucchini, large and diced

- Sea salt and black pepper to taste

- 1/2 Cup of 2% milk

- 1/4 Teaspoon of nutmeg

- 1 Tablespoon of lemon juice, fresh

- 1/2 Cup of cheddar, grated

- 8 Ounces uncooked farfalle pasta

Directions:

1. Get out a skillet and place it over medium heat, and then heat up the oil. Attach in your garlic and cook for a minute. Stir often so that it doesn't burn. Add in your salt, pepper, and zucchini. Stir well, and cook

covered for fifteen minutes. During this time, you'll want to stir the mixture twice.

2. Get out a microwave-safe bowl, and heat the milk for thirty seconds. Stir in your nutmeg, and then pour it into the skillet. Cook uncovered for five minutes. Stir occasionally to keep from burning.

3. Get out a stockpot and cook your pasta per package instructions. Drain the pasta, and then save two tablespoons of pasta water.

4. Stir everything together, and add in the cheese, and lemon juice and pasta water.

Nutrition Facts Per Serving:

Calories: 813.76 kcal

Total Fat: 34.79 g

Carbs: 99.71 g

Sugars: 13.74 g

Protein: 27.15 g

Sodium: 577.9 mg

Potassium: 1000 mg

Phosphorus: 500 mg

Spicy Cabbage Dish (Healthy)

Note: To make this recipe, a Slow Cooker is needed; alternatively, a Dutch oven or any heavy-duty pot with a good lid will work.

Preparation Time: 10 minutes

Cooking Time: 4 hours

Servings: 4

Ingredients:

- 2 yellow onions, chopped

- 10 cups red cabbage, shredded

- 1 cup plums, pitted and chopped

- 1 teaspoon cinnamon powder

- 1 garlic clove, minced

- 1 teaspoon cumin seeds

- 1/4 teaspoon cloves, ground

- 2 tablespoons red wine vinegar

- 1 teaspoon coriander seeds

- 1/2 cup water

Directions:

1. Combine cabbage, onion, plums, garlic, cumin, cinnamon, cloves, vinegar, coriander, and water to your Slow Cooker.
2. Stir well.
3. Place lid and cook on LOW for 4 hours.
4. Divide between serving platters.
5. Serve.

Nutrition Facts Per Serving:

Calories: 219.48 kcal

Fat: 1.38 g

Carbohydrates: 51.05 g

Protein: 3 g

Phosphorus: 183 mg

Potassium: 1350 mg

Sodium: 113.37 mg

Extreme Balsamic Chicken (Healthy)

Preparation Time: 10 minutes

Cooking Time: 25 minutes

Servings: 2

Ingredients:

- 3 boneless chicken breasts, skinless

- 2 tbsp. almond flour

- 1/3 cup low-fat chicken broth

- 1 teaspoon arrowroot

- 1/4 cup low sugar raspberry preserve

- 1 tablespoon balsamic vinegar

Directions:

1. Slice chicken breast into bite-sized pieces and season them with seeds.
2. Dredge the chicken pieces in flour and shake off any excess.
3. Set a non-stick skillet and place it over medium heat.
4. Add chicken to the skillet and cook for 10 minutes, making sure to turn them halfway through.
5. Remove chicken and transfer to a platter.

6. Add arrowroot, broth, raspberry preserve to the skillet and stir.

7. Stir in balsamic vinegar and reduce heat to low; stir-cook for a few minutes.

8. Transfer the chicken back to the sauce and cook for 10 minutes more.

9. Serve.

Nutrition Facts Per Serving:

Calories: 546 kcal

Fat: 35 g

Carbohydrates: 11 g

Protein: 44 g

Phosphorus: 120 mg

Potassium: 117 mg

Sodium: 85 mg

Enjoyable Green Lettuce and Bean Medley

Note: To make this recipe, a Slow Cooker is needed; alternatively, a Dutch oven or any heavy duty pot with a good lid will work.

Preparation Time: 10 minutes

Cooking Time: 4 hours

Servings: 2

Ingredients:

- 3 carrots, sliced

- 1 cup great northern beans, dried

- 1 garlic clove, minced

- 1/2 yellow onion, chopped

- Pepper to taste

- 1/4 teaspoon oregano, dried

- 2.5 ounces baby green lettuce

- 2 1/2 cups low sodium veggie stock

- 1 teaspoon lemon peel, grated

- 1 1/2 tablespoon lemon juice

Directions:

1. Combine beans, onion, carrots, garlic, oregano, and stock to your Slow Cooker.
2. Stir well.
3. Set the lid and cook on HIGH for 4 hours.
4. Add green lettuce, lemon juice, and lemon peel.
5. Stir and let it sit for 8 minutes.
6. Divide between serving platters and serve!

Nutrition Facts Per Serving:

Calories: 570.63 kcal

Fat: 2.17 g

Carbohydrates: 110.17 g

Protein: 33.13 g

Phosphorus: 700 mg

Potassium: 1500 mg

Sodium: 145.82 mg

Cauliflower and Dill Mash (Healthy, Low Caloric)

Note: To make this recipe, a Slow Cooker is needed; alternatively, a Dutch oven or any heavy-duty pot with a good lid will work.

Preparation Time: 10 minutes

Cooking Time: 5 hours

Servings: 3

Ingredients:

- 1/2 cauliflower head, florets separated

- 2 tbsp. + 2 tsp. cup dill, chopped

- 3 garlic cloves

- 1 tablespoon olive oil

- Pinch of black pepper

Directions:

1. Add cauliflower to Slow Cooker.
2. Add dill, garlic and water to cover them.
3. Place the lid and cook on HIGH for 5 hours.
4. Drain the flowers.
5. Season with pepper and add oil, mash using potato masher.

6. Whisk and serve.

Nutrition Facts Per Serving:

Calories: 42.74 kcal

Fat: 3.03 g

Carbohydrates: 3.55 g

Protein: 1.26 g

Phosphorus: 28.84 mg

Potassium: 185.43 mg

Sodium: 18.19 mg

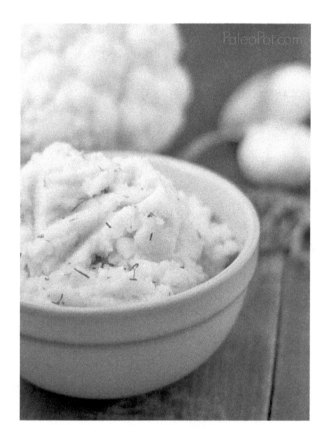

Peas Soup

Preparation Time: 10 minutes

Cooking Time: 10 minutes

Servings: 2

Ingredients:

- 1/2 white onion, chopped

- 1/2 tsp. olive oil

- 1/2 quart veggie stock

- 1 egg

- 1 1/2 tablespoons lemon juice

- 1 cup peas

- 1 tablespoons parmesan, grated

- Salt and black pepper to the taste

Directions:

1. Take a pot and heat 1 tsp. oil over medium-high heat
2. Then, add the onion and sauté for 4 minutes.
3. Attach the rest of the ingredients except the eggs, bring to a simmer, and cook for 4 minutes more.
4. Add whisked eggs, stir the soup, cook for 2 minutes more, divide into bowls and serve.

Nutrition Facts Per Serving:

Calories: 264 kcal

Fat: 7.2 g

Fiber: 3.4 g

Carbs: 33 g

Protein: 17 g

Sodium: 800 mg

Potassium: 600 mg

Phosphorus: 300 mg

Basil Zucchini Spaghetti

Preparation time: 1 hour and 10 minutes

Cooking time: 10 minutes

Servings: 4

Ingredients:

- 1/3 cup coconut oil, melted

- 4 zucchinis, cut with a spiralizer

- 1/4 cup basil, chopped

- A pinch of sea salt

- Black pepper to taste

- 0.25 cup walnuts, chopped

- 2 garlic cloves, minced

Directions:

1. In a bowl, mix zucchini spaghetti with salt and pepper, toss to coat, leave aside for 1 hour, drain well and put in a bowl.
2. Warmth up a pan with the oil over medium-high heat, add zucchini spaghetti and garlic, stir and cook for 5 minutes.

3. Add basil and walnuts and black pepper, stir and cook for 3 minutes more.
4. Divide between plates and serve as a side dish
5. Enjoy!

Nutrition Facts Per Serving:

Calories: 287 kcal

Fat: 27 g

Fiber: 3 g

Carbs: 8 g

Protein: 4 g

Sodium: 75 mg

Phosphorus: 110 mg

Potassium: 117 mg

Cauliflower Rice and Coconut

Preparation Time: 20 minutes

Cooking Time: 15 minutes

Serving: 4

Ingredients:

- 3 cups cauliflower, riced

- 2/3 cups full-fat coconut milk

- 1-2 teaspoons sriracha paste

- 1/4- 1/2 teaspoon onion powder

- Salt as needed

- Fresh basil for garnish

Directions:

1. Take a pan and place it over medium-low heat.
2. Combine all of the ingredients and stir to mix well.
3. Let cook for about 5-10 minutes, making sure that the lid is on.
4. Then, remove the lid and keep cooking until there's no excess liquid.
5. When the rice becomes creamy, serve it.

Nutrition Facts Per Serving:

Calories: 225

Fat: 19 g

Carbohydrates: 4 g

Protein: 5 g

Sodium: 60 mg

Phosphorus: 150 mg

Potassium: 600 mg

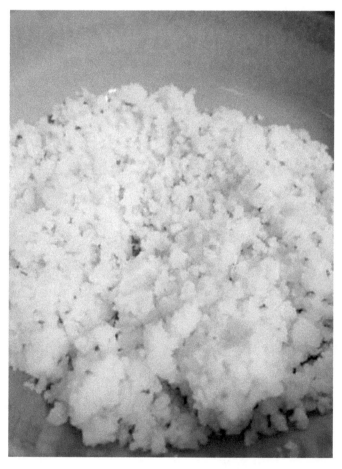

Kale and Garlic Platter

Preparation Time: 5 minutes

Cooking Time: 12 minutes

Serving: 2

Ingredients:

- 1/2 bunch kale

- 1 tablespoon olive oil

- 2 garlic cloves, minced

Directions:

1. Remove kale stem and cut into bite-sized pieces.
2. Then, set a large-sized pot and let heat olive oil over medium heat.
3. Add garlic and stir for 2 minutes.
4. Add kale and cook for 5-10 minutes.
5. Serve!

Nutrition Facts Per Serving:

Calories: 121 kcal

Fat: 8 g

Carbohydrates: 5 g

Protein: 4 g

Sodium: 81 mg

Potassium: 900 mg

Phosphorus: 220 mg

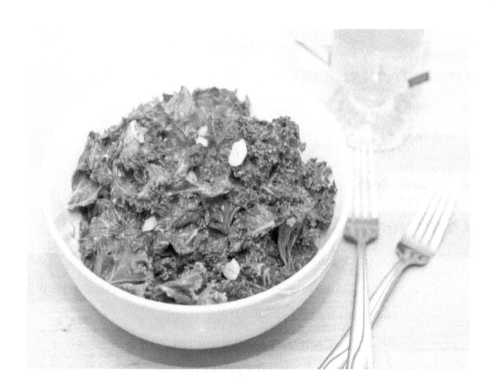

Healthy, Blistered Beans and Almond

Preparation Time: 10 minutes

Cooking Time: 20 minutes

Serving: 2

Ingredients:

- 1/2 pound fresh green beans, ends trimmed

- 1 tablespoon olive oil

- 1/8 teaspoon salt

- 1 tablespoon fresh dill, minced

- Juice of 1/2 lemon

- 1/8 cup crushed almonds

- Salt as needed

Directions:

1. First, preheat your oven to 400 F.
2. Take a bowl and add in the green beans with olive oil and salt.
3. Then, take a large-sized sheet pan and spread them on it.

4. Roast for 10 minutes and stir nicely, then roast for 8-10 minutes more.

5. Remove it from the oven and keep stirring in the lemon juice alongside the dill.

6. Top it with crushed almonds, some sea salt, and serve.

Nutrition Facts Per Serving:

Calories: 98 kcal

Fat: 7.83 g

Carbohydrates: 7.57 g

Protein: 1.86 g

Sodium: 236 mg

Potassium: 161 mg

Phosphorus: 33 mg

Cucumber Soup (Low Caloric)

Preparation Time: 10 minutes

Cooking Time: 0 minutes

Serving: 2

Ingredients:

- 1 tablespoon garlic, minced
- 2 cups English cucumbers, peeled and diced
- 1/4 cup onions, diced
- 1/2 tablespoon lemon juice
- 1 cup vegetable broth
- 1/4 teaspoon salt
- 1/8 teaspoon red pepper flakes
- 1/8 cup parsley, diced
- 1/4 cup Greek yogurt, plain

Directions:

1. Take a blender and attach the listed ingredients (except 1/4 cup of chopped cucumbers).
2. Blend until smooth.

3. Divide the soup amongst four servings and top with extra cucumbers.

4. Serve.

Nutrition Facts Per Serving:

Calories: 53 kcal

Fat: 1.26 g

Carbohydrates: 8.77 g

Protein: 2.33 g

Sodium: 238.19 mg

Potassium: 273 mg

Phosphorus: 67 mg

Eggplant Salad

Preparation Time: 10 minutes

Cooking Time: 50 minutes

Serving: 3

Ingredients:

- 2 eggplants, peeled and sliced

- 2 garlic cloves

- 2 green bell pepper, sliced, seeds removed

- 1/2 cup fresh parsley

- 1/2 cup egg-free mayonnaise

- Salt and black pepper

Directions:

1. First, preheat your oven to 480 F.
2. Then, take a baking pan and add the eggplants and bell pepper
3. Bake the vegetables for about 30 minutes and flip them after 20 minutes.
4. Then, take a bowl and add baked vegetables and all the remaining ingredients.
5. Mix well.
6. Serve.

Nutrition Facts Per Serving:

Calories: 196 kcal

Fat: 10.8 g

Carbohydrates: 13.4 g

Protein: 14.6 g

Sodium: 310 mg

Potassium: 1100 mg

Phosphorus: 121 mg

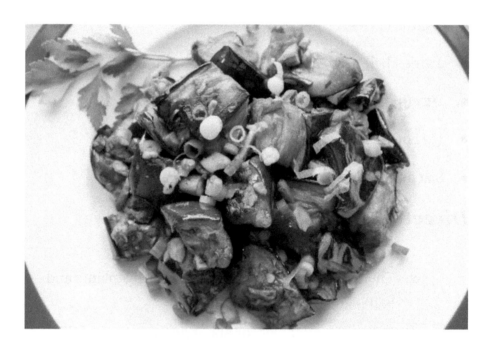

Cajun Crab (Low Caloric)

Preparation Time: 10 minutes

Cooking Time: 10 minutes

Serving: 2

Ingredients:

- 1 lemon, fresh and quartered

- 3 tablespoons Cajun seasoning

- 2 bay leaves

- 4 snow crab legs, precooked and defrosted

- 1 tsp. golden ghee

Directions:

1. Set a large pot and fill it about halfway with water and salt.
2. Then, bring the water to a boil.
3. When water is boiling, squeeze the lemon juice into the pot and toss in the remaining lemon quarters.
4. Add bay leaves and Cajun seasoning.
5. Then, season for 1 minute.
6. Add crab legs and boil for about 8 minutes (make sure to keep them submerged the whole time).

7. Melt ghee in the microwave and use it as a dipping sauce.

8. Serve.

Nutrition Facts Per Serving:

Calories: 49.71 kcal

Total Fat: 0.39 g

Carbohydrates: 0.65 g

Protein: 10.39 g

Sodium: 771.66 mg

Potassium: 125.93 mg

Phosphorus: 123 mg

Mushroom Pork Chops

Preparation Time: 10 minutes

Cooking Time: 40 minutes

Serving: 3

Ingredients:

- 8 ounces mushrooms, sliced

- 1 teaspoon garlic

- 1 onion, peeled and chopped

- 1 cup egg-free mayonnaise

- 3 pork loins

- 1 teaspoon ground nutmeg

- 1 tablespoon balsamic vinegar

- 1/2 cup of coconut oil

Directions:

1. Take a pan, add the coconut oil and let heat it up over medium heat.
2. Then, add mushrooms, onions, and stir well.
3. Cook for 4 minutes.
4. Add pork loins and season with nutmeg, garlic powder, and let brown both sides.

5. Bring the pan to the oven and bake for 30 minutes at 350 F.
6. Transfer pork loins to plates and place aluminum foil on top to keep them warm.
7. Take the same pan and place it over medium heat.
8. Add vinegar, mayonnaise over the mushroom mixture and stir for a few minutes.
9. Drizzle sauce over pork loins.
10. Serve.

Nutrition Facts Per Serving:

Calories: 400 kcal

Total Fat: 18.39 g

Carbohydrates: 1.4 g

Protein: 30g

Sodium: 91.71 mg

Potassium: 158.89 mg

Phosphorus: 73.72 mg

Caramelized Pork Chops

Preparation Time: 5 minutes

Cooking Time: 30 minutes

Serving: 2

Ingredients:

- 2 pounds pork chops

- 1 tsp. salt

- 1 tsp. pepper

- ½ tsp. olive oil

- 2 ounces green chili, chopped

- 2 tablespoons chili powder

- 1/4 teaspoon dried oregano

- 1/4 teaspoon ground cumin

- 1 garlic clove, minced

- 1 onion, sliced

- ½ glass of water

Directions:

1. Coat your pork chops with 1/2 teaspoon of pepper and 1/2 teaspoon of seasoning salt, chili powder, oregano and cumin.
2. Then, take a skillet and heat 1/2 tsp. oil over medium heat with the garlic.
3. Brown your pork chops on each side.
4. Add water and onion to the skillet.
5. Cover and lower the heat, simmer it for about 20 minutes.
6. Turn your loins over and add the rest of the pepper and salt.
7. Cover until the water evaporates and the onions turn a medium brown texture.
8. Remove the chops from your skillet.
9. Serve with some onions on top!

Nutrition Facts Per Serving:

Calories: 500 kcal

Fat: 19 g

Carbohydrates: 4 g

Protein: 27 g

Sodium: 91.71 mg

Potassium: 153.89 mg

Phosphorus: 73.72 mg

Mediterranean Pork

Preparation Time: 10 minutes

Cooking Time: 35 minutes

Serving: 2

Ingredients:

- 2 pork chops, bone-in

- ½ tsp. salt

- pepper to taste

- 1/2 teaspoon dried rosemary

- 1 1/2 garlic cloves, peeled and minced

Directions:

1. First, preheat your oven to 425 F.
2. Season pork chops with salt and pepper.
3. Place them in a roasting pan and add rosemary and garlic.
4. Bake for 10 minutes.
5. Lower heat to 350 ° F and roast for 25 minutes more.
6. Slice pork chops and divide on plates.
7. Drizzle pan juice all over
8. Serve.

Nutrition Facts Per Serving:

Calories: 335 kcal

Fat: 17.42 g

Carbohydrates: 1.52 g

Protein: 40.48 g

Sodium: 668 mg

Potassium: 566 mg

Phosphorus: 351 mg